DAPOXETINE MED GUIDE

Understanding Dapoxetine Its Mechanism, Uses, and Impact on Premature Ejaculation (PE) Treatment

DR JONATHAN PAUL

Table of Contents

- CHAPTER ONE 3
  - Introduction 3
- CHAPTER TWO 6
  - What is Premature Ejaculation? 6
- CHAPTER THREE 13
  - Mechanism of Action 13
- CHAPTER FOUR 16
  - Dapoxetine Dosage 16
- CHAPTER FIVE 20
  - Efficacy (How Well Does it Work?) 20
- CHAPTER SIX 23
  - Common Side Effects 23
- CHAPTER SEVEN 27
  - Uses of Dapoxetine 27
- CHAPTER EIGHT 30
  - Contraindications 30
- CONCLUSION 35

CHAPTER ONE

Introduction

A short-acting selective serotonin reuptake inhibitor (SSRI), dapoxetine is mostly prescribed to men for the treatment of premature ejaculation (PE). It functions by raising serotonin levels in the brain, which can lengthen ejaculation times and increase control over the process. The first oral drug created especially for PE is dapoxetine, which is sold under several trade names, including Priligy.

Inhibiting the serotonin transporter causes a rise in serotonin activity in the postsynaptic cleft, which is the mechanism of action of dapoxetine. Because of its well-established importance in the ejaculatory process, this neurotransmitter's enhanced availability has the potential to postpone ejaculation.

Dapoxetine is usually taken in doses of 30 or 60 mg, one to three hours prior to planned sexual activity. It is not advised to take it more than once per 24 hours. Several clinical trials have assessed the effectiveness and safety of dapoxetine, showing that it can considerably enhance patient-reported outcomes related to control over ejaculation and sexual satisfaction as well as the Intravaginal Ejaculatory Latency Time (IELT).

Dapoxetine frequently causes headache, nausea, dizziness, and diarrhea as adverse effects. The intensity of these adverse effects is usually mild to moderate, and they tend to get better with continuing use. Dapoxetine, however, should not be taken by people who have specific medical conditions, such as serious cardiac issues, or who are taking drugs that interact with SSRIs, such as thioridazine and monoamine oxidase inhibitors (MAOIs).

Although dapoxetine cannot treat PE, it does offer men who have the ailment a useful therapeutic choice. It's crucial for anyone thinking about taking dapoxetine to speak with a medical expert to find out if it's the right course of action for them given their medical background and present state of health.

CHAPTER TWO
What is Premature Ejaculation?

Men often experience premature ejaculation (PE), which is defined as ejaculating earlier than anticipated, either before or soon after penetration, causing discomfort for one or both partners. Though the precise duration can vary, it is often characterised by the incapacity to postpone ejaculation for longer than around one minute following vaginal penetration. PE can be acquired as a secondary or lifelong main condition.

Lifelong PE, which is frequently related to genetic or neurological causes, starts with a person's first sexual experiences and lasts the entirety of their lives. After a time of normal sexual functioning, acquired PE can occur. It may be linked to underlying medical diseases, psychological causes, or relationship problems.

While the precise causes of PE are still unknown, a number of risk factors have been found. Atypical hormone levels, inflammation or infection of the prostate or urethra, and aberrant ejaculatory system reflex action are examples of biological causes. Psychological elements, such as interpersonal issues, depression, worry, and stress, can also be quite important.

Beyond the realm of sexual activity, PE can have a negative impact on one's self-esteem, induce anxiety, and exacerbate interpersonal problems. Significant emotional and psychological distress can be experienced by men with PE and their relationships.

A comprehensive medical history and physical examination are usually required for the diagnosis, with special attention paid to psychological and sexual history. Premature Ejaculation Diagnostic Tool (PEDT) questionnaires are among the many tools used to evaluate the disease.

PE can be treated using behavioral strategies like the squeeze or stop-start methods as well as counseling or therapy to address underlying psychological problems. Medications such as dapoxetine and topical anesthetics are examples of pharmaceutical treatments that are frequently used to manage symptoms. The greatest outcomes are frequently achieved by combining various therapeutic modalities, which relieve symptoms and increase sexual satisfaction for both couples.

Open communication with a healthcare professional is essential for the effective management of PE in order to determine the best treatment plan based on each patient's unique needs and circumstances.

How Does PE With Dapoxetine Work?

A selective serotonin reuptake inhibitor (SSRI) called dapoxetine was created especially to treat men's premature ejaculation (PE). It works by raising the brain's serotonin levels, which helps improve control over ejaculation and postpone the ejaculatory response.

Dapoxetine works primarily by blocking the serotonin transporter, a protein that helps serotonin get reabsorbed into presynaptic neurons from the synaptic cleft. Dapoxetine prolongs the action of serotonin on postsynaptic receptors by increasing the concentration of the neurotransmitter in the synaptic cleft through inhibiting this transporter. One neurotransmitter that is essential for controlling mood and inhibiting ejaculation is serotonin. It is thought that better ejaculatory control and delayed ejaculation are related to increased serotonin activity.

Dapoxetine is appropriate for use on-demand because it absorbs quickly and achieves peak plasma concentrations in 1-2 hours after oral dosing. 30 mg or 60 mg should be taken one to three hours prior to plan sexual activity. Dapoxetine's effects wear off rather rapidly due to its short half-life of roughly 1.5 hours, which reduces the possibility of long-term negative effects that are usually connected with SSRIs.

Dapoxetine has been shown in clinical trials to markedly increase the Intravaginal Ejaculatory Latency Time (IELT), or the amount of time it takes to ejaculate following vaginal penetration. It has also been demonstrated to enhance patient-reported outcomes for sexual satisfaction, control over ejaculation, and a decrease in interpersonal challenges and emotional anguish related to PE.

Dapoxetine frequently causes headache, nausea, dizziness, and diarrhea as adverse effects. With sustained use, these side effects—which are typically mild to moderate—tend to go away. People with serious cardiac issues or those taking drugs that could negatively interact with SSRIs should not use Dapoxetine.

For men with PE, dapoxetine is a useful therapy choice that can improve both sexual performance and enjoyment. To guarantee its safety and effectiveness based on unique health profiles, it should be used under the supervision of a healthcare provider.

CHAPTER THREE
Mechanism of Action

A selective serotonin reuptake inhibitor (SSRI) called depoxetine was created especially to treat premature ejaculation (PE). Its main mode of action is based on modifying serotonin levels, which are important neurotransmitters that control mood, anxiety, and the ejaculatory reflex.

A multitude of brain processes, including sensory input, central processing, and muscular output, are involved in the intricate ejaculatory process. This mechanism is significantly inhibited by serotonin, especially in the central nervous system (CNS). The serotonin transporter (SERT), a protein that facilitates serotonin's reabsorption from the synaptic cleft back into the presynaptic neuron, is inhibited by dapoxetine.

Dapoxetine improves serotonergic neurotransmission by raising serotonin levels in the synaptic cleft through inhibiting SERT. A delay in ejaculation results from an increase in serotonin availability at postsynaptic receptors in brain and spinal cord regions involved in the ejaculatory reflex. The specific regions affected include the spinal ejaculation generator and the lateral paragigantocellular nucleus, both of which are essential for ejaculation regulation.

Dapoxetine is a medication that can be used as needed because of its quick absorption and short half-life of about 1.5 hours. It takes

1-2 hours to reach peak plasma levels, which is in perfect timing for sexual activities. This pharmacokinetic profile reduces long-term negative effects linked to long-term SSRI usage, which is a benefit.

Dapoxetine successfully lengthens the Intravaginal Ejaculatory Latency Time (IELT) and enhances overall ejaculation control, according to clinical research. In addition to delaying ejaculation, the increased serotonergic activity also lessens stress and anxiety, which can worsen PE.

Notwithstanding its advantages, dapoxetine has various negative effects that should be taken into account, including headache, nausea, and dizziness. It should also not be used in specific groups of people, such as those who have serious cardiovascular problems. Patients should speak with medical professionals to find out if dapoxetine is a good fit for their particular situation.

CHAPTER FOUR

Dapoxetine Dosage

Dapoxetine is usually used as needed and is indicated especially for the treatment of premature ejaculation (PE) in men. Dapoxetine should be started at a dose of 30 mg, taken one to three hours prior to planned sexual activity. The dosage may be raised to a maximum of 60 mg based on each patient's effectiveness and tolerability. It is crucial to remember that taking dapoxetine more than once in a 24-hour period is not advised.

Dapoxetine's quick absorption means that it can reach peak plasma concentrations in one to two hours, which is in line with its recommended use right before sexual activity. By restricting exposure to the medication when it is not needed, this timing ensures that the drug is effective when needed and lowers the possibility of negative effects linked to prolonged SSRI usage.

Dapoxetine gives the user freedom by being taken with or without food. However, in order to lower the possibility of unpleasant gastrointestinal side effects, it is advised to take it with a full glass of water. Additionally, patients are recommended to abstain from alcohol while using dapoxetine because it may raise their risk of experiencing adverse effects like sleepiness, syncope, and dizziness.

Dapoxetine frequently causes nausea, headaches, dizziness, diarrhea, and sleeplessness as adverse effects. Most of the time, these side effects are low to moderate in intensity and often go away as you continue to take the product. However, people should speak with their healthcare practitioner if adverse symptoms worsen or continue.

Men who use drugs that negatively interact with selective serotonin reuptake inhibitors (SSRIs), such as monoamine oxidase inhibitors (MAOIs) and some antipsychotics, or who have serious cardiovascular disorders, such as heart failure or conduction abnormalities, should not take dapoxetine. Since SSRIs might affect mood and behavior, it is also not advised for people who have a history of serious psychiatric illnesses.

To find out if dapoxetine is a good treatment option, a complete medical evaluation by a healthcare provider is necessary before beginning. To reduce risks and provide the best possible therapy of premature ejaculation, this also entails an assessment of the patient's medical history, current medications, and general health status.

CHAPTER FIVE

Efficacy (How Well Does it Work?)

The intravaginal ejaculatory latency time (IELT) and total sexual pleasure have been demonstrated to be considerably improved by dapoxetine, an effective treatment for premature ejaculation (PE). Its effectiveness is well supported by clinical trials and research, which makes it a worthwhile choice for men with PE.

The main way to assess dapoxetine's effectiveness is to look at how it affects IELT, or the interval between vaginal penetration and ejaculation. Men taking dapoxetine in clinical trials usually had a three- to four-fold rise in IELT over baseline readings. For instance, dapoxetine therapy frequently increased the average IELT of men, who had an ejaculatory delay of about one minute, to three or four minutes. This was a significant improvement.

Dapoxetine has also been demonstrated to improve ejaculation control and lessen the discomfort and interpersonal challenges related to PE. Results from patient surveys show improved overall relationship quality, less anxiety, and increased happiness with sexual activity. Given that they address both the psychological and physical aspects of PE, these advancements are crucial.

Due to its short half-life and quick start of action, dapoxetine can be used as needed, offering flexibility and reducing long-term negative effects linked to long-term SSRI use. Men can use the medication as needed rather than continuously every day by taking it one to three hours before they want to engage in sexual activities.

Real-world research, in addition to clinical trials, have validated the efficaciousness and safety profile of dapoxetine. With continued use, the side effects, which might include headaches, nausea, and dizziness, usually subside to a mild to moderate degree. But in order to maximize benefits and reduce side effects, following the recommended dosage and timing is essential.

All things considered, dapoxetine provides many men with PE with a well-tolerated and efficient treatment option that enhances their quality of life and sexual performance. However, because each person's response is unique, speaking with a healthcare provider is crucial to figuring out the best course of action given your unique needs and medical problems.

CHAPTER SIX
Common Side Effects

Although it works well to treat premature ejaculation (PE), dapoxetine has a number of negative effects. The majority have mild to moderate degrees of severity and tend to get better with repeated use. But it's important for users to know about these possible side effects and to see a doctor if they have any negative responses.

Dapoxetine frequently causes nausea, headaches, dizziness, diarrhea, and sleeplessness as adverse effects. The most common negative effect that users report experiencing is nausea, which affects a considerable percentage of consumers. Headache and dizziness are also frequent and might interfere with day-to-day activities, especially during the early phases of treatment. Though less often, diarrhea and sleeplessness can nevertheless happen and can be uncomfortable.

A few less frequent but more dangerous adverse effects are mood swings, hypotension (low blood pressure), and syncope (fainting). Orthostatic hypotension, or a sharp drop in blood pressure upon standing, is typically associated with syncope and hypotension. This may cause lightheadedness, vertigo, or even fainting. To reduce this risk, users are encouraged to get up gently from seated or lying down situations.

Although they are less prevalent, mood swings including despair and anxiety can happen when using dapoxetine. Dapoxetine affects mood and behavior since it is a selective serotonin reuptake inhibitor (SSRI). Individuals who have previously experienced mood disorders ought to utilize dapoxetine cautiously and under constant medical supervision.

Because of the risk of syncope and other cardiac events, dapoxetine should not be used in people with serious cardiovascular problems, such as heart failure or conduction abnormalities. Additionally, it is not advised for those on drugs like thioridazine, antipsychotics, or monoamine oxidase inhibitors (MAOIs) that have negative interactions with SSRIs.

When taking dapoxetine, alcohol should be avoided as it can aggravate adverse effects like syncope and dizziness. When recreational drugs or other chemicals that alter serotonin levels, like MDMA or LSD, are combined with dapoxetine, the risk of serotonin syndrome, a potentially fatal illness, increases.

Dapoxetine is generally well tolerated, however in order to guarantee safe and efficient use, users should be aware of any side effects and speak with their healthcare professional.

Treatment outcomes for premature ejaculation can be optimized and side effects can be managed with the support of a healthcare provider and regular follow-ups and open communication.

CHAPTER SEVEN

Uses of Dapoxetine

Premature ejaculation (PE) is a frequent sexual disorder in men that is mostly treated with dapoxetine. PE is characterized by ejaculation that happens sooner than expected, either before or immediately after penetration, causing distress for one or both partners. Effective therapy is crucial since PE can have a major negative influence on one's interpersonal relationships, self-esteem, and quality of life.

The purpose of the selective serotonin reuptake inhibitor (SSRI) dapoxetine is to raise serotonin levels in the brain. One of the main factors preventing ejaculation is serotonin. Dapoxetine works by prolonging its activity at the synaptic cleft by inhibiting the absorption of serotonin. This helps to delay ejaculation and enhance control over the time of ejaculation.

Dapoxetine enhances overall control over ejaculation and increases the intravaginal ejaculatory latency time (IELT) considerably, according to clinical trials. The average IELT can rise three or four times for many men, which results in increased sexual satisfaction and decreased PE-related anxiety. Better control over ejaculation, a reduction in psychological anxiety, and an improvement in interpersonal skills are frequently observed alongside this improvement in IELT.

When using Dapoxetine, it is usually taken one to three hours prior to planned sexual activity. 30 mg is the suggested starting dose; however, based on each patient's efficacy and tolerability, this can be increased to 60 mg. It is not advised to take it more than once in a 24-hour period. Convenient and helpful in lowering the possibility of adverse effects linked to long-term SSRI use is this on-demand dosage.

Common adverse effects, which are usually mild to moderate and tend to go away with sustained use, include headache, nausea, dizziness, and diarrhea. Though uncommon, serious adverse effects can include mood swings, hypotension, and syncope (fainting). Men with serious cardiovascular diseases or those on drugs that may negatively interact with SSRIs should not take dapoxetine.

CHAPTER EIGHT
Contraindications

Dapoxetine should not be used in a number of certain groups because of possible hazards and harmful interactions. To guarantee the safe and efficient use of the medicine for the treatment of premature ejaculation (PE), it is imperative to comprehend these contraindications.

Heart-Related Disorders

Due to its tendency to raise blood pressure and heart rate, dapoxetine should be avoided by those with serious cardiovascular diseases. Those who have:

Severe cardiac conditions

Heart attack

The arrhythmias' past

Recent heart attack, or myocardial infarction

Unchecked blood pressure

Dapoxetine can make these illnesses worse, increasing the risk of dangerous cardiac events including arrhythmias, syncope (fainting), or even a worsening of heart failure.

Dapoxetine has negative interactions with a number of drug types, including:

Monoamine Oxidase Inhibitors (MAOIs): When dapoxetine and MAOIs are used together, serotonin syndrome, a potentially fatal illness marked by agitation, hallucinations, a fast heartbeat, and erratic blood pressure, can occur. It is necessary to wait a sufficient washout period (usually 14 days) before beginning dapoxetine after discontinuing an MAOI.

Thioridazine: Because of the higher risk of severe cardiac arrhythmias, thioridazine, an antipsychotic drug that can lengthen the QT interval, should not be taken with dapoxetine.

Other SNRIs and SSRIs: The risk of serotonin syndrome may rise if dapoxetine is taken in combination with other SNRIs or serotonin-norepinephrine reuptake inhibitors (SNRIs). There should be a washout interval while alternating these drugs.

Behavioral and Psychological Health

Dapoxetine usage should be cautious in people with a history of psychiatric problems or unstable mental health situations. SSRIs have the ability to affect behavior and mood, which may exacerbate underlying medical issues or have detrimental psychological impacts.

Getting older and overall health

Because there is insufficient information about the safety and effectiveness of dapoxetine in these age ranges, it is not advised for use by those who are younger than 18 or older than 65. Additionally, because dapoxetine may alter medication metabolism and clearance, patients with hepatic disease should use caution or avoid using it completely.

It is critical that medical professionals perform a comprehensive evaluation of the patient's medical history, current medications, and general health status prior to starting dapoxetine therapy. This assessment aids in determining possible contraindications and reduces the risks related to using dapoxetine.

To promote safe treatment management and maximize outcomes for PE, patients should always disclose to their healthcare practitioner any current medical conditions or drugs.

CONCLUSION

A selective serotonin reuptake inhibitor (SSRI) called dapoxetine is authorized to treat men's premature ejaculation (PE). The following highlights its application, mode of action, effectiveness, and important factors:

Mechanism of Action: Dapoxetine increases serotonin levels in the brain by blocking the serotonin transporter. By improving serotonergic neurotransmission, this helps postpone ejaculation and gives you more control over when to ejaculate.

Efficacy: Men usually have a three- to four-fold increase in intravaginal ejaculatory latency time (IELT) compared to baseline, with clinical trials demonstrating dapoxetine to considerably increase IELT. Together with this improvement come less PE-related distress and improved ejaculation control.

Dosage and Administration: One to three hours prior to planned sexual activity, dapoxetine is taken as needed. 30 mg is the suggested starting dose; however, based on each person's response and tolerability, this can be increased to 60 mg. It is not advised to take it more than once per 24 hours.

Adapaxetine side effects can include headache, nausea, dizziness, diarrhea, and sleeplessness. They usually range from mild to moderate and get better with repeated use. Treatment-related serious adverse effects, including mood swings and syncope (fainting), must be closely monitored.

Contraindications: People who use MAOIs or thioridazine, have a history of psychiatric illnesses, or have substantial cardiovascular disorders (such as severe heart disease or uncontrolled hypertension) should not take dapoxetine. Patients who are older than 65 years old or who are less than 18 should not use it.

Drug Interactions: Dapoxetine may cause serotonin syndrome or other severe side effects when combined with MAOIs, thioridazine, and other SSRIs/SNRIs. To prevent negative interactions, patients should disclose to their healthcare practitioner all prescriptions, including over-the-counter medications and vitamins.

Patient considerations: Based on the patient's health status and prescription regimen, a thorough medical evaluation is required prior to initiating dapoxetine in order to determine suitability. During treatment, patients must completely follow all recommended dosages and guidelines and abstain from alcohol.

www.ingramcontent.com/pod-product-compliance
Lightning Source LLC
Chambersburg PA
CBHW072049230526
45479CB00009B/327